I AM LOVE

I am love, I am kind
I am giving but
I have limits

I am love, I am unique
I am human and
I have flaws

I am love, I am patient but
I have boundaries

I am love, I am compassion
I am understanding and

I have a journey, A journey of love
A journey with others,
A journey home

ABOUT ME

My life changed suddenly after I was diagnosed with an auto-immune disease. It was not a life-threatening disease, but it resulted in several hospital visits, strong medication and put my life on hold. It impacted every aspect of my life emotionally, physically, mentally, and financially. It drained me of my energy and enthusiasm, as it tested me beyond my mental and physical limits. After several years, the disease took everything from me, but I refused to give it my hope. I hung to it tightly, my hope for a way back.

My hope began to materialise when I came to realise that it was only me that was holding the power for my own healing. I realised that I had to stop waiting for a magic cure. I had to stop waiting for someone else to save me and I had to save myself. I started to accept that the old life was gone but I could make the most and best of what a new life could be. I decided that I would heal for me and not for anyone else. I decided that I was going to be empowered to rise, despite being powered to fall.

I began changing my thoughts and my mind to be as positive as they could be. I practiced daily gratitude for all I had, and I dedicated as much time to my mind as to my physical body. As my thoughts began to change, I gained a new perspective on my situation. I began to realise that the disease itself was not a life sentence for negativity and because of it I was learning how to live a new life. It was stopping me in my tracks to slow down, to listen and to pay attention to the world around me. A world I had forgotten and a world I had ignored.

The disease was giving me a new appreciation for life and I realised that, rather than drowning in sorrow, I could use my experience to help others who are also going through a difficult time. I began to understand that it happened for a reason, and that by helping others I could further embrace my own life journey. I could embrace my own healing. I could be empowered by it and empower others.

I wrote this book to help you to become empowered with whatever it is you might be struggling with. My hope is that this book will help you to gain a new perspective and a new belief that life can be good again and that you deserve life to be good again.

This book is dedicated to all of you going through a difficult time, either physically or mentally. It is dedicated to each of you who start each day with a new hope that healing is possible. It is for you to know that you do not have to suffer alone, and that you are universally supported and eternally held in love. It is for you to know no matter how dark your days have been, that brighter ones lie ahead.

I hope this book supports you on your own journey back to finding your true health, wealth, happiness, and love. I have written this book from my heart to yours.

INTRODUCTION

There is a true beauty at the heart of each one of us. We all have a unique and beautiful soul that shines brightly. It was God's gift to us, our beautiful soul. It allows us to see the beauty in others. It allows us to forgive others for their mistakes. It is the place from which we can love eternally and unconditionally.

This part of us is always there, but due to life circumstances, it can diminish. We can become lost within ourselves and we can lose the power of our light. We can lose our ability to love others, love ourselves and we find it impossible to forgive and move past the hurt. We become stuck in past regrets, resentments, and thoughts. We torture ourselves with what-ifs and try to change something that is no longer possible to change. It is over, but we struggle to move on. We struggle to release and let go. We struggle to embrace the new.

Each day is a new chance to start again, but many of us do not take this chance. We can wake up with a negative mindset, and not long out of bed, we absorb large amounts of negative news. We may be working in places we do not want to work, as we feel pressure to pay the bills and we can become victims in our own life stories. It can become impossible to see the way out and we can continue like this until something eventually breaks.

The break can come as an opportunity for change, or a life sentence to our own prison. It can come as a chance to reassess and revaluate where we are, and where we are going. It can offer us a chance to look around and find the beauty again. The beauty in the small and simple things all around us. The beauty in the things that we once took for granted. The beauty within us and among others.

When we break, we can take this chance to rebuild our lives and live as we were meant to, as a beautiful and loving soul. We can give gratitude in whatever way the break has come. It may have come a lesson. It may have come to redirect us on our path. When we are broken, we should not be afraid to ask for help to put it all together again. It is only in love, that we can rise again.

We all take an individual journey of love, forgiveness and learning how to let go. On our journey, we can be broken time and time again. We can be tested beyond our limits and we can fall without anyone to catch us.

Even when we lose the power of our light, it never gets extinguished. It remains, waiting for us to reignite it again with love from within. It is never too late for us to start again. To start a new journey, and a new life. It is never to late for us to shine our light and love brightly as we were born to do.

CHAPTER 1

HEALTH: IN MIND AND BODY

Our health gives us the ultimate freedom in achieving what we want in life. It gives us the freedom to do whatever it is we want, go wherever we want and be whatever it is we want. It gives us freedom of choice, freedom of movement and freedom to financial independence.

To be healthy is to be free. Free to choose our career, and our path. Free to be independent of others. Free to stand on our own two feet. Our health is the biggest gift of all, yet it can easily be the first thing we take for granted. We might never give it a second thought that each morning we can get out of bed, walk around, dress ourselves and put food on the table.

When we take a moment to stop, we can give gratitude for the health that we do have and for the health of our loved ones. We can stop and think about how blessed we are to still have the health of our parents and grandparents. We can think of those not so fortunate.

Achieving good health comprises of both mind and body. We should never judge a person's true health from the outside alone. A person may look healthy physically but, on the inside, struggle emotionally. On the other hand, a person with a physical disability can have a strong, happy, and resilient mind.

To be physically healthy is only part of the picture. Both mind and body are connected, and our health can only benefit from working on both. We can work towards a healthy mind by choosing positive thoughts and we can work towards a healthy body by making positive decisions.

The mind is much more powerful than we will ever comprehend. The mind stores the memories caused by our life experiences and over time positive and negative memories begin to accumulate. The memories we store are the building blocks to our belief system. Our belief system impacts every decision we make, and our belief system impacts our decision to choose the positive.

Like attracts like, and for every negative thought we think, more will come but with each positive thought we intercept it with, we can attract more positive thoughts in its place. We can only change our thought pattern by becoming aware of it. When we become aware of the pattern, we are in complete control to change it.

If we decide to change the pattern, we can actively intercept negative thoughts as they arise. We can stop them in their tracks before they gain momentum and replace them with the positive. When we change the thought, we change the belief. By changing the mind, we change the body, and we change our health.

WEALTH: RESPONSIBILITY

By blaming others, we avoid taking responsibility for our own mistakes and life circumstances. Despite what has gone before us, our future is yet to be told. Our future is always in our hands and we are ultimately responsible for our own happiness. When we blame another person for our unhappiness, we hand them over the power to our life and we hand them the key to our own happiness.

It is easy to use the hurt caused by others as a reason to be unhappy and it is easy to avoid the truth. The truth sits in front of us and the truth sits within us. We know it is only us that can create our own happiness, but somehow it is easier to blame others when we do not have the life we want. It is easier to bury our heads in the sand and avoid taking responsibility.

Our life circumstances and happiness are never dependent on another person. It starts and ends with us and it starts with responsibility. Another can come into our life and add to our happiness, but it is our responsibility to set the foundation first. We are responsible for planting our own roots firmly in the ground. Others can come along and help us grow and as we grow, some branches will fall but new ones will come in their place.

There is no other that can come along and change our life circumstances for us. We are what we have created, and we have created what we are, with our thoughts, our beliefs, our decisions, and our own free will. When we take our own personal responsibility for what has happened until now, we also take full responsibility to choose what happens next and we take back the power to our own life.

In responsibility we become empowered. In responsibility we choose how we react and respond to the actions of others. In responsibility we focus our efforts on what is in our hands to change. In responsibility we realise that we cannot control the actions of others, but only how we respond.

If we respond negatively and in blame towards another, we hand them the control to our happiness and our circumstances. If we choose to respond positively, we can learn something from the situation and move forward in our lives without blame and anger towards others.

When we start taking responsibility for our own life, the actions of others cannot impact our inner state, and cannot interfere with our inner happiness. When we forgive others for their mistakes, we free ourselves of the hurt, and free ourselves from them.

No matter what the hurt caused, it cannot be changed, and it cannot be undone. We can only ever choose what happens next. We always hold the choice to take our power back from others and choose a positive life. We always have the choice to rise in responsibility.

HAPPINESS: GRATITUDE I

We can live our lives today in critical and negative thought patterns because of what we observed growing up. Despite having enough, we can find reasons to complain about not having enough. We create ongoing negative patterns when we think about what we do not have. We have an opportunity to shift our perspective when we start to practice gratitude for what we do have.

A prayer of thanks before eating can shift our perspective from a place of scarcity to a place of abundance. From a place of complacency to a place of gratitude. We can always offer gratitude for the food that is in front of us and take a moment to think of those who cannot afford to eat or for those that are too sick to eat.

Instead of looking for the one thing to complain about, we can look for things to be thankful for. Instead of criticising those around us, we can face and change our own shortcomings. Instead of being perfectionists, we can start to see the beauty in human flaws. When we start to look for the beauty, we can find it.

As soon as we start to shift our perspective to a place of gratitude, we shift our mind to the positive. As soon as we decide that we are done with complaining, our happiness can flow. As soon as we decide to break the negative cycle, our world can change before our very eyes.

In making the decision to be positive and replace our negative thought patterns, we will watch those around us change too.

They know that their negative behaviour is not acceptable to us anymore and that our tolerance for it is gone. As we begin to change our thoughts, the people in our life will change too. New people will come into our life that reflect our new thoughts and our new patterns.

When we start choosing new thoughts and expressions of gratitude, we will see the immediate mental benefits of choosing a positive mind. Our stress levels will reduce, as our minds become clearer and we feel a weight lifted from our shoulders.

We can all actively start to find things to be grateful for, and when we do, we can speak of them out loud and to others. We can write them down and begin sentences with "Isn't it great because" or "I am so thankful for". It might be new language for us at first but with ongoing repetition and determination to change, it will soon become more natural and frequent for us.

The more we give thanks, the more reasons we have to be thankful. The more positive we are, the more positivity will flow into our life. When a negative thought arises, it is up to us to question it and to stop it. It is up to us to replace it with a thought of gratitude or appreciation. The more we allow gratitude to flow, the more happiness will flow.

LOVE: IS ETERNAL

Life is temporary by nature. Nothing lasts forever. The seasons change, our appearance changes, people come and go from our lives and our children grow up and leave home. Life changes in every moment. This is good to remember in a difficult time, as it too shall pass. It too is temporary.

Love is different. True love is not temporary. True, unconditional love is eternal. When someone we have loved is no longer physically with us, our love for them remains and gets left behind. It is not temporary. It lingers long after they are gone. We can close our eyes at any moment and remember how it feels to still love them. Love survives everything else.

As love is eternal, a love physically lost is still a love worth having. When we remember how it felt to be loved or to love, it is the most beautiful and nurturing feeling for our soul. We should never regret loving someone, even if they have left our life. Their love has taught us something, and that love has been a gift. If only for a short time, we can still cherish the time we had with that person. It is always worth opening our heart, even if the person is no longer with us.

When someone we love decides to walk away from our life, it is natural to feel hurt and rejected. Rejection is an extremely hard emotion to process as we spend most of our lives looking to be accepted in love. When someone we love rejects us, we question our own self-worth, and what we did wrong. We have given them our heart and we are left heart broken. We cling on to the hope that they will return and love us again.

When love comes and it is temporary or conditional, we must let it go. This type of love is not worth having and is not real love. As this type of love is dependent on life circumstances changing, it will change too as life changes. Since change in our lives is inevitable, this type of love cannot last the test of time. When we find our true love, it will support change and it will support us through the change.

If someone can stop loving us because of life circumstance, then their love for us was based on external circumstance. Their love was never based on us. There are some that do not know true love, and they might never know. Their love will always be temporary and superficial. Their love will always seek excuses to walk away and there will never be anything we can do to turn conditional love into unconditional.

A relationship will go through love highs and lows. Sometimes, walking away from someone we love and creating physical space is needed. Sometimes, we need distance to gain a different perspective, to gain a new appreciation for what we do have and to reassess our future. We should always allow someone we love to have that space. We should always be patient with love. If our love is true love it will find its way back to us, brighter and better than before.

CHAPTER 2

HEALTH: MOVEMENT AND STILLNESS

It is easy to make excuses as to why we are not as healthy as we could be. Typically, our excuses are because of time and money. Long-term wellness starts by removing these excuses and choosing to commit to making positive lifestyle changes. Even if the change is small to start, it is better than no change at all. Small changes can be made regardless of time or money. It never has to cost us money to move, and we can all make the time for the right food choices.

There are many things available to us to improve our health that are at hand. A walk outside, yoga stretches, a long hot bath, a cold shower, self-massage and deep breathing are free and accessible to us at any time. These practices help us physically, but more importantly they help us mentally. They change our state of mind and slow down the nervous system to go back into balance.

We will feel lasting and positive benefits by practicing a wellness routine daily, even if only for twenty minutes a day. Once we start to feel the benefits, we may find that we want to increase the time and might even start to say no to the things that someone else can do. By actively pursuing our wellness routine, we actively learn how to prioritise ourselves and our own needs.

If we start to incorporate mindfulness into our lives each day, we may notice that we become less overwhelmed by everyday stress. When we clear our minds, we are naturally more balanced to face the ongoing pressures and stresses of life. If we set up a space in our home for our mindfulness practice we can go there whenever we feel the need to recharge and reset.

Mindfulness is a simple practice to bring us back into our natural balance. Mindfulness includes meditation which can help us to quieten the mind and bring us into a state of awareness in the present moment. When we are in a meditative state, we come into the present moment by our breath. When we in a meditative state, we become aware of our physical body in the present.

Our minds benefit from stillness, but our bodies are built to move. Exercise achieves both states by bringing the mind into the present moment, as it moves the body. Movement keeps our bodies strong and stillness keeps our minds clear. When we move, we allow new energies to come into our bodies. When we are still, we allow old thoughts move out from our minds.

Making time for our daily wellness routine is something we must actively pursue and prioritise. There is plenty of information available to us for choosing how we practice our daily wellness routine. It is available at our fingertips. We can access it anytime, we can move anytime, and we can be still anytime. We can bring wellness into our lives anytime. We can choose today.

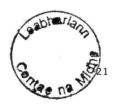

WEALTH: THE GREATEST GIFT

A child is a gift given to us from the eternal place of love. A child is a blessing from above. When born, a child embodies what love is. A child knows nothing else but love when it comes into this world. A new-born child is the purest form of love that we will know.

As parents, we must protect our children from harm. We must nurture and teach them how they give and receive love to themselves and to others. As parents, we must show our children forgiveness for their mistakes and kindness through understanding.

A child by its very nature is creative and explorative, and there are some that may find it difficult to concentrate for long periods. As parents and teachers, we are in the ultimate place of responsibility to our children to show them patience in their learning.

Each child will have their own unique gifts and abilities and we should freely encourage them for their uniqueness. Regardless of what their abilities are, continuous words of praise will help build their confidence and self-belief. When we remind them of the love that we have for them, they will learn to speak loving words to themselves.

A child should not feel inadequate to others academically and we must remain mindful of placing our own expectations on our children. We should never place pressure on our children in achieving certain grades or compare our children with others.

If a child is asked the right questions, they will come up with the right answers and in the process, they will build their self-confidence. We should always support a child when they make mistakes and encourage them to try again in their own time and space. We should give them the independence they need to grow and allow them to freely express their thoughts and feelings without judgement.

If we speak openly and often of our love to a child, they will know and speak of love for themselves and for others. By forgiving them for their mistakes, they will forgive others. By accepting them for who they are and not who we want them to be they will accept themselves.

We cannot place our own worries or fears on our children, and we must free them from our own emotional baggage. We must hold them in a place of safety, support, freedom, and love. A child is the greatest gift of all and a gift from above. A gift of love in its original, unaltered form. A gift to remind us of our own inner love in its purest form.

HAPPINESS: FORGIVENESS

When we learn how forgive, we learn how to be free. When we forgive others, we free our hearts from the hurt and disappointment caused by others. Forgiveness does not mean that we must accept poor behaviour or put up with less than we deserve. When we forgive, we recognise that human error and imperfection exist. Forgiveness gives us the permission to release the hurt caused by others.

When we hold negative feelings towards another, we hold this energy somewhere inside our body. This negative energy is not good for us. It is heavy and it is draining. By holding it, we replay it in our mind over and over again and continue to suffer emotionally and mentally for someone else's mistakes. This negative energy blocks the positive coming in. We must make a conscious effort to release the negative to experience the positive.

When we replay the hurt caused by others, it reinforces the negative effect on the mind and body. It causes us unnecessary and ongoing stress and we gain nothing from burning our precious life energy on past mistakes. We need our energy to live fully in the now and it is only in forgiveness that we can stop burning. It is only in forgiveness that we move to the positive and the present.

Whatever anyone has done to hurt us, we must remember that they did so because they are hurting themselves and they did not know any better. There are times when we are suffering that we can make mistakes, act out and hurt others unintentionally.

An act of unintentional hurt is part of life and part of love. There is nobody that will escape life without experiencing some form of human hurt. It is part of our life experience and growth. We hurt others and they hurt us. Life is complicated at times and we can hurt without even realising it.

We cannot live our life in this moment if we cannot release the past. We can only move into the present by making peace with the past as it was, and not how we wished it to be. Making peace with our past involves accepting all that was or was not, good and bad. It involves looking back without judgement or regret. We must let it be and we must let it go.

Sometimes we need forgiveness ourselves. We may not even realise that we need forgiveness. We may be holding guilt, shame, or regret deep within us. It comes a time when we must let go and forgive our own mistakes. The less we hold of our past, the more we can receive of our future.

The act of forgiveness will set our heart free and the act of compassion will set our soul free. Forgiving is an act for self. Compassion is an act for others. At its depth, forgiveness is love. Love yourself enough to forgive. Love yourself enough to be free.

LOVE: CHOOSE LOVE

Love is an ongoing process in life, and love is our own personal journey of growth. Love is the strongest and most beautiful feeling of all when we feel it from deep within our being. Love is the most eternal feeling of all. We were born in love and we were born to love. That is our core and that is our centre.

Attracting love is something we must actively work at. We need to actively seek it and be open to receiving it. Love, when searching for it, must start from within. It is sitting there in our soul, waiting for us to remember it from when we first came into this world.

Love is our natural state of being, but we can forget this along our life path. When we move away from our centre, we can move back to it through awareness that if this was our state once, then it can be our state again. Through awareness, we can connect to this place inside of us that radiates love.

If we were not shown love regularly as a child, we have moved away from our centre. If we did not speak of love regularly as a child, it can be uncomfortable to speak loving words towards ourselves and to others. If we did not experience loving affection from our parents, we might not freely give affection to our own children.

When we were young, we were taught that showing love makes us weak, when in fact it makes us stronger. It binds us together like no other and it makes us resilient. It allows us to heal. When we know how to love, and love from the heart, our love allows us to forgive others.

By choosing love over hate, we create the best life for ourselves and for those around us. By choosing love each, time, the negative actions of others do not disrupt our lives as we remain grounded by love. By choosing love, we choose not react to another's mistakes. We can just let it be. We can let it go.

Love is always worth the work and worth the effort. When all is said and done, it is only love that will remain, and it is only love that will get us through. It is only love that can give us the strength when we need it the most. It is only in love that we see the light again. Love for ourselves and love for others.

When we remember how to love ourselves, we in turn set good expectations for ourselves. These expectations set in motion the belief that we deserve good things. This belief will manifest itself and become our reality. When we forget how to love ourselves it will have the opposite effect.

We have nothing to lose and everything to gain by remembering and choosing to love ourselves again. Instead of waiting for those around us to love us, we can love ourselves. If others have forgotten how to love, we may be a lifetime of waiting. At the end we will realise we could have just felt love from within and love from our centre.

CHAPTER 3

HEALTH: BACK TO BASICS

Eating a well-balanced and varied diet is an essential part of being well, feeling well and having sustained energy levels. Eating a well-balanced diet gives us the physical benefits of looking well but more importantly it gives us the mental benefits of feeling well. When we establish a healthy attitude towards food, we give our children good and lasting habits that they can pass onto future generations.

The world of what to eat and how to eat has become so complicated in recent years. It has become big money. It has become a long list of complex and conflicting information. We can get lost in all the information available. To eat and be well, we could simply go back to basics.

We could go back and look at what our grandparents did. They had simple, healthy, varied diets and they ate from the land. They kept sugar and processed food to a minimum and they prioritised home cooking. All types of food were enjoyed in moderation and mealtimes were important times that were shared as a family.

Our grandparents would typically offer a prayer of thanks before eating and had an appreciation for the food they would work hard to harvest. They ate with the cycles and ate most of their food in its natural state. They understood and appreciated the natural flow of the cycles and the land.

Our grandparents lived basic lives when it came to their food and lifestyle choice, but this simplicity served them well. There was little or no fuss made when it came to food, and they had a deep appreciation for all that they had. All members of the family contributed to the work of the household and there was no such thing as a free meal.

In our grandparent's time, there was a sense of community and a sense of support through that community. Each would be willing to lend a hand and each would be willing to accept the help. They would look out for each other and made time for each other. No matter how busy their day was, there was always time for tea and always time to talk.

Their daily movement included working on the land or working in the home and they spent little time sitting. They used natural herbs and remedies where possible and medication played a minimal part. They took a well-rounded approach to their lifestyle, and as a result lived long and happy lives.

There is much to learn from this time and how our grandparents lived. There is much to be gained from going back to basics in our own lives. There is much appreciation to be found in the simple life. There is much to pass on to future generations, from past generations and from their long, happy, and healthy lives.

WEALTH: CRITICAL THINKING

There are times when we can be our own worst enemy. We give ourselves a hard time unnecessarily because of our own low self-esteem and self-worth. We all have an inner critic inside us somewhere. Some days it will be louder than others. When we start listening it, we become aware of how loud it is. Awareness is the first step to intercepting it and replacing it with a different voice.

We seldom stop and praise ourselves for our small achievements, yet we are quick to judge ourselves easily for our mistakes. When we are critical towards ourselves, we can mirror this onto others, and we can mirror this onto the world. We can become an inner and outer critic of almost anything and nothing ever seems good enough.

We need to actively remind ourselves that we are doing ok and so is everyone else around us. We should actively praise ourselves and others. We should freely give out compliments. The more we can self-praise, the more we can praise others. The more we look for the good in ourselves, the more we will see the good in others. The truth is, everyone is doing or trying their best and some days it is harder than others. Some days it is a struggle, and we can never really know someone else's struggle.

Criticism can come easy to us, but it achieves nothing. There is no good that can ever come out of being critical towards another. The act of criticising will only serve to negatively impact another's self-esteem and confidence. The act of criticising is finding fault for the sake of finding fault. It is putting someone down instead of raising them up.

Critical patterns can be changed through awareness. When we become aware of our thoughts and patterns, we can start to question our pattern, and question what kind of energy we are creating with our critical thinking. We can challenge ourselves to think of something to praise instead. We can challenge ourselves to look for the positive over the negative. We can challenge ourselves to choose praise and encouragement every time.

During difficult periods in our lives, it is easy to fall victim to critical thinking. Life has become hard and life is not fair. It is only natural when we are faced with a negative situation to feel despair. The natural response when faced with a negative situation is to think negatively. By reacting negatively, we compound the situation.

When we become a victim to negativity and criticism, we build our own prison wall. With each negative thought, we lay a brick for our wall. With each brick we build, it becomes harder and harder to see our way out. It is only by consciously shifting to a more positive place of praise and encouragement, that we can start to move the bricks and let the light in again to our very own freedom.

HAPPINESS: RISING ABOVE

When someone hurts us, we are free to choose how we overcome the hurt. We can become angry by it or we can walk away from it. We can become empowered or consumed by it. We can become stuck in it or be free from it. We can sink or rise above it. The choice is always ours.

There may be a lesson we can learn when someone hurts us. There may be something that we can take forward as a positive to counteract the negative action of the hurt. There may even be a new boundary that we can put in place. By taking positive action, we remain in control of our future and how someone else will treat us. We always hold the power to walk away so that the same hurt is not repeated.

When we remind ourselves that we are always in control of how we react when others hurt us, we can empower ourselves to rise above the hurt. By taking a positive out of a negative situation, we can turn the original action around on its head. We can turn it around in our favour. Sometimes, the action required may just be about doing nothing at all and giving ourselves the time and space to heal before we face life again.

We may become wiser and stronger because of the hurt that another has caused us. It may result in us having healthier and more balanced relationships in the future. It may result in us prioritising our own needs before meeting the needs of others.

We should try to acknowledge and process the hurt at the time that it is caused. Even if it is difficult to face, if ignored, it will get stored as anger or resentment somewhere in the body. When it is stored, it will raise its head again. When we give it a voice, we can release it.

Any form of physical or mindful exercise can help us to process and release the hurt caused and stored. Exercise can help us to release any negative blocked energy in our minds or bodies. When we quiten our minds and stop overthinking, we may gain some new perspective and clarity on the situation. By choosing to be mindful, we choose to support our mental and emotional well-being.

We can process and release the hurt by talking. In talking, we can release what we are holding, acknowledge what has happened and move forward with the positive. In moving forward, we rise above the situation for our greater good. We learn a lesson and we take that forward in our favour.

If we cannot find another to listen, we can write about it instead. We can write a letter or keep a diary. Any act of expression is encouraged, to release our thoughts and our feelings. We should always find time to find out what supports our mental health. We should always find time to rise past and above the hurt.

LOVE: IT MUST BREAK TO REBUILD

There are times in life when it will get too much, when we will fall apart or watch those around us fall apart and we feel powerless to help them. There are times when life as we knew it can change without warning, and we are left wondering how we will ever cope or love again. We can lose a loved one suddenly. They can be taken from us, or they may have chosen to walk away.

In these moments, we can go into a state of shock and a state of grief. We may become overwhelmed not knowing how we will cope. As we are faced with the ultimate heartbreak of loss or grief, we are left with a hole in our heart, and a piece of us is missing. We feel empty inside. We have so many unanswered questions. There are no words to describe our loss, we are just broken.

In these moments, we need to show ourselves as much kindness, compassion, patience, and love as we can. We need to take it as slow and as easy as we can. We need to take each day as it comes. We need not look too far into the future. We can only take each day at a time and look at getting through as best as we can, as gently as we can.

We need to allow ourselves as much space and time to heal and remove any timelines for doing so. We need to be allowed to sit with and be in our sadness. We need to just be. For some, the healing may last a lifetime. We may slowly be able to move on and rebuild our lives without them, but we will never forget a lost love.

No one will ever be able to replace them.

It is sometimes in those darkest, loneliest moments, that we will find our true inner strength and courage. We may find that somewhere inside us lies the ultimate human strength of getting through. At our lowest point we may find the truth and strength that lies within our soul.

In these moments, we might look to prayer to help us through. Prayer is sometimes the most powerful of all. A prayer from the heart for help never goes unanswered. It may not always be answered in the way we had hoped, but it will be answered in some form.

The help needed in getting through can come from above and can come from God. The feelings of loneliness and despair can be lifted through prayer alone. If we can believe it, we are never truly alone and there is always an angel nearby and ready to help us. Our guardian angel never leaves us and there is always a God full of love who has created us.

In our lowest and darkest moments, our inner self, our outer world and everything we knew will be broken. It will all be taken away and we will have to start again. We will have to rebuild the new. A new life and a new you. As time passes, we may slowly be able to let go of the old and step into a new you. A new stronger you. A new beautiful you.

CHAPTER 4

HEALTH: A CHANGE
OF SCENE

We can get caught up in the routine of everyday life. We are always busy, there is always somewhere to be and there is never enough time. Frustrations may soon arise when there is no end in sight of a never ending to do list. We spend so much time chasing time, and in doing so we can lose sight of what is important. We can lose sight of ourselves.

We all need a change of scene of some kind from our everyday lives. Making the time to break away from everyday life is something we should actively pursue and actively prioritise. When we take the time away from our routine, we can recharge and reset our minds and our bodies. Taking a break of any kind can offer us a chance to gain a new perspective and a new mindset.

When we change our setting and surrounding, it is good for the soul and good for the mind. When we break our routine, we give ourselves a chance to reassess, reset and regain a much-needed perspective and direction in our life. The more we can switch off from our busy lives, the more we can listen to where we are going.

When we set a date for a break away, we have something to look forward to and work towards. We have an end in sight. As we change our surroundings, we change how we think, change how we feel and create a space to release the old and welcome in the new.

When possible, we should take a break when we can on our own.

When we remove ourselves from the home and make time for ourselves, we teach our family a valuable lesson. We show them the importance of self-care and independence. We teach them to cope without us and appreciate us more in our absence.

We can break from our routine when we walk into nature and switch off our phones and connections. When we switch off what is going on in the outer world, we can begin to pay attention to what is going on inside. When we make the time to look within, we can listen and learn how to prioritise ourselves and our own needs.

Sitting in nature, brings us back into the present moment. When we sit and observe all that is around us, we can start to appreciate the world that has been given to us. When we observe animals in their natural environment, it can remind us about the beauty and the simplicity of life. It reminds us of the natural flow of life. It reminds us to appreciate the interconnectedness of our world and the interconnection of each one of us. It is only by changing our scene, that we can change what we see.

WEALTH: LEARNING TO LISTEN

If we mastered the skill of active listening, we could master success. Lasting success and building a business is usually achieved because of a team effort. To lead a team successfully we must know how to influence others. This skill is achieved not by talking but by listening. Active listening.

Active listening involves both listening and understanding. When we listen with sincerity and compassion, we can understand each other. When we understand each other, we remove judgement and can respect each other. With respect for each other, we can achieve great things together.

When we take a sincere interest in what another person is saying, they will feel valued, appreciated, and important. When someone feels important, they feel that their work is equally important. They will want to put in the effort and energy to succeed for themselves and for others because they have felt appreciated.

A good listener will give another the space to talk and ask the right questions so that another can arrive at their own conclusions. A good listener knows that another already knows the answer to solving their own problems, but all they need is a good sounding board to figure it out.

When someone is speaking, it is important to refrain from interrupting to give our own point of view. It is important to wait until they are finished, consider their opinion, and give a constructive opinion in the context of what has been said.

An opinion with a few words can be more valuable than a never-ending story about our own life. Active listening does not involve bringing the conversation back to self. Active listening is not waiting on the side-lines to interrupt. Active listening is not waiting to hear our own voice. It takes patience and practice to learn the simple act of just listening and being present.

If someone has a different opinion to us, we must remember not to take it personally or feel the need to defend our own position. There is no reason to be offended because someone else has a different point of view. We must remember that difference is inevitable and because of life experience or circumstance, others will have another view of the world.

We can always listen and accept another point of view even if we do not agree with it. Accepting it does not make one person wrong and one right. Acceptance means understanding. We have all come from a different place in life and we are all going in a different direction. We all have a unique perspective from where we are standing. When we learn to listen to each other from where we are standing, we can stand together despite our differences.

HAPPINESS: THE TIME IS NOW

Waiting for life to be perfect to start doing means that we will end up waiting forever. The timing will never be perfect. Life can never be perfect. There will always be something standing in our way. There will always be that one excuse not to start.

The timing will never be exactly right to start doing or becoming. There will always be something or someone standing in our way. There will always be that story we have told ourselves and others as to why it must be put it off to some point in the future. By putting it off, we avoid facing our fears. Our fear of failure and our fear of what we are truly capable of achieving.

The reality is that life is short, and life will not wait. Our lives are precious and none of us know how much time we have left. There will come a time when we need to stop waiting and excusing. There will come a time to start looking for the hundred reasons why we should face the world as it is today.

Deep down we know what our life purpose is. Deep down we know that by starting we might just change our world. We might even change the lives of others. Deep down we have allowed fear to take a hold and we are denying ourselves and the world our unique gifts and abilities.

We are only fooling ourselves with all the excuses. The excusing prevents us from doing and achieving what we were born to do. We have created our own story behind the excuses, and we have started to believe in it. It comes a time when we must start to question that story. It comes a time to start facing our fears.

Our fears hold us back more than we realise. We hold them subconsciously, so we might not even realise they are there. We might not realise the strong hold they have over us. They are the root cause for us ignoring our life purpose. They are the root cause for us hiding.

When fear exists, it is difficult to tune into what our heart really wants as it blocks off the vital communication between head and heart and stands firmly in its way. Fear takes on a voice of its own and this voice can fill our head with doubt. This voice will eat away at our self-belief.

When we start to become aware of our fears, we can start to question them one by one and begin to understand where they have come from. By questioning them, we can overcome them. When we overcome them, we remove the block that is holding us back.

It is only by doing that we can fully face and conquer our fears. We can finally prove to ourselves how capable and how brilliant we really are. We can knock the fear on the head. We can rationalise the irrational. We can look directly at our fears and decide that the time is now, and the time is right.

LOVE: FORGIVE TO KNOW LOVE

Relationships will come in and out of our lives and teach us some form of lesson, be it good or bad. Each relationship will teach us something about ourselves and who we are becoming. Each one will force us to face parts of ourselves we would rather leave asleep. We may even be taught the same lesson time and time again until the lesson is learned.

The pattern of attracting the same people into our lives will continue until we face the lesson to be learned. When someone loves us, they teach us love. When someone hurts us, they teach us forgiveness. Forgiveness at its depth is love, and it comes from the same place. In forgiveness, we connect to a place in our soul. The lesson from others is always about connecting to our soul.

Love will come to us easier than forgiveness. When someone hurts us, we take it personally. We take it to our heart, and we can hold it there as hate. If we were to shine love on the hurt, we could release it, we could let it go, and we could open the part of us that is compassion. That part of our soul.

There are few in life that will set out intentionally to cause us harm. For most people, actions of hurt are generally caused by the unconscious. Their hurtful actions reflect what is going on inside for them. They are struggling inside and releasing their hurt in hurting others.

An action of hurt must be consciously handed back to the other person for them to process. It cannot be left sitting with us as hate in our heart. By shining a light on it and sending it back to them with love and compassion, we break the cycle of hurt. We learn the lesson, and we connect to our own internal place of love.

It is important for us to forgive so that we can learn how to trust another again. When we hold onto the hurt, we form a negative view of the world. We hold onto the fear that we can be hurt again, and we find it difficult to trust again. If we cannot trust again, we cannot genuinely love again. We cut ourselves off from receiving new love again, in its fullness.

When we forgive others and love again, it will be better than we could have ever imagined. It will flow naturally and flow fast. We all deserve to be loved. We all deserve to find our true love. We all deserve to find a place to receive unconditional love.

It is only in forgiveness we can find the true meaning of love. By forgiving, we can remember that we are all eternally held in love and in light. We are love and so are others. The act of forgiving reminds us of our love, and the act of compassion reminds them of theirs. We should always seek to be reminded and to remind others. We should always choose to forgive in love.

CHAPTER 5

HEALTH: A DOG'S LIFE

A dog will bring an abundant amount of unconditional love into our life. They have no limits when it comes to loving us. A dog is the most loyal friend we will ever have. It is an unbreakable bond, the bond between man and dog. A bond that lasts a lifetime.

When a dog comes into our life, they can come at a time of great personal need. They can come to bring us enormous healing by their presence and their love. They need no words to show us their love. When they hand us their paw or lick our face, we know that we are held in love by them.

A dog is completely forgiving. They do not hold on to anything and start each day anew. They start each day with enormous amounts of energy, enthusiasm, and joy. They live for the moment and in the moment. They bring us into the moment when we are around them.

A dog can make us laugh and melt our heart from a place that we never knew of before. A puppy brings new and vibrant energy to any home. Their innocence and curiosity for life is impossible not to be drawn into. Their sense of fun and enthusiasm for life is infectious.

A dog will bring us outside much more than we had bargained for. It is hard to ignore their face when it comes to walking time. It is hard to ignore their simple need to be out in the fresh air running around. Although an initial effort, there is never a walk that we regret with our dog.

A dog will not use the excuse of bad weather to be out and about. They enjoy the rain as much as the sun in the sky. They smell every blade of grass in sight, curious of everything that nature has to offer. They bring the same curiosity back to us. They bring us back time and time again.

A dog loves meeting new people regardless of who they are or where they meet them. They run to strangers, and greet them with affection, and with love. They are always looking for an excuse to receive affection and attention from others and they are never offended if another ignores them.

A dog can teach us much about health and about life. They can teach us the importance of food, exercise, sleep and play. They can show us how to start each day anew and to let go of what has gone before. They can show us how to love unconditionally and to be present in each moment.

A dog reminds us of the simple but happy life. They provide us with reminders of the simplicity of walking and appreciating nature. They remind us of the power of giving and receiving love freely. They remind us of the simplicity and power of unconditional love.

WEALTH: DO UNTO OTHERS

"Do unto others as you would have them do unto you" is a powerful statement worth reflecting on. This statement has the power to change us. It has the power to change the world. When we treat others as we would expect to be treated, we could remove the inequality and injustice in our world. We could start to live aligned to each other, in love.

It comes easy to us, to do the best for our children, and for those that we love but it might not come as easy to us when it comes to a stranger that we encounter. It might be a stranger that needs our love the most, but instead, we have given it to a family member because they are labelled family.

We have separated ourselves from each other into circles of family, friends, and neighbours. We have chosen to separate ourselves by borders, religion, and politics. Even with manmade separation, we remain interconnected at a higher level. We all come from and are going to the same place. We are interconnected more than we will ever know.

When we start thinking and acting as a collective, powerful things are possible. When we start thinking beyond our circles and borders, we can change the world. When we start thinking of the needs of others as we would our own family, the world can change for the better of mankind and future generations.

The recent outbreak of a global virus has shown us how much we are all interconnected. We are all in it together and we can only get through it together. We must act as a collective. We must think of ourselves and of others. We must think of family and of strangers. We must act to protect the lives of the most vulnerable and we must act in the best interests of everyone. Everyone we know and everyone we do not know.

When faced with these challenging times, there will be those who do not participate in the collective. There will be those that bring it back to themselves, and those that act out of self-interest. There are those that will use the situation to create fear and hate in others. As a collective, we cannot allow the selfish actions of others to steer us off the collective path to a greater good. We must remain steadfast in our shared belief that together we stand stronger. That together, we support and love another.

In the face of adversity, we can become unified in one, and unified in love. The virus has taken down the borders that we have created. It has taken down the circles that we have created, and it has shone a light on the inequality in the world that we have created. We were never intended to be separated by these manmade creations, so by "doing unto others", we are doing on to the collective and doing on to ourselves. When we do good for others, we in fact do good for ourselves.

HAPPINESS: FAILURE IS AN OPTION

We hold the fear of failure within and perceive it as a negative outcome. This fear can control us, and we can give up easily when we initially fail at learning something new. We feel that failure is a direct reflection on our personal ability, and failure causes us to doubt our own capability to achieve our goals. When we fail, we worry what others will think of us. We worry how others will judge us.

Failure is only the opportunity to learn what could have be done differently so that we can do it better the next time. Like solving a maths equation or problem solving, it can take numerous attempts to come up with the solution but in each attempt, we move closer to the answer. In each attempt we increase our chances of success and we will finally arrive at the solution. In giving up after the first attempt, we remove our chance of success. We remove our chance at life.

When we learn a new skill or stop an old habit, failure will be part of the process. Each time we fail, we can take a new piece of learning forward. The learning will eventually add up to a positive result in achieving our goals. When we continue in the face of failure, it is only ever a matter of time before we succeed. With resilience and persistence, we will achieve our success.

If we were to achieve what we wanted to first time around, we would have learnt little in the process. It is only in failure that we can learn to grow. There will always be something to learn from our failure and it is always the journey that counts. The result is only the reward for making it to the end.

We could start to see failure as a chance to know more than those around us, which increases our chances of success in the future. Each time that we have tried, we have acquired additional know how that will help us the next time we try. There is no successful person that has achieved success without failure and in the process, they have mastered the skill of getting up and trying again. They have mastered the skill of life.

If we do not pick ourselves up from failure, there will be no one else to pull us up. There will be no one else to achieve our dreams for us. We must stand on our own in the face of failure. We must stand when it is not the outcome we expected or when we are disappointed with the result. It is in these times that we are tested.

There will come a day that even in the face of failure, we decide to do it anyway and achieve what we want out of life. This is a powerful moment to embrace. It is in this moment, that we accept and own that failure is an option and by owning it we cannot fear it. When we do not fear it there is nothing or nobody standing in our way of the life that we want or our dreams that we dare to dream.

LOVE: KNOW YOUR OWN HEART

Highly opinionated people can be extremely irritating when we meet them or work with them. Sometimes we are related to them. They have an opinion on everything and anything and they feel the need to express it often and regularly whether they are asked to or not.

They feel the need to tell others how to live their lives, yet often it is their own lives that need sorting. They feel the need to interfere in the lives of others when it is their own life that needs attention. By interfering in the lives of others, they avoid facing up to their own problems.

A self-opinionated person will never be open to learning from another. They have an answer for everything and are closed off to another point of view. There is nothing to learn from them, and them from you as they already seem to know it all. There will always be some who like the sound of their own voice. There will always be some who feel the need to interfere.

When faced with the interfering opinions of others, we must know our own minds and our own value. We must know our own heart. We can overcome this interference by mastering our own self-belief and connection to heart. When we connect to this place, we back ourselves, our decisions and let that of others pass on by. We let it pass on by without giving it any form of attention. It should never be because of others or their opinions that we move away from our life path and purpose. If another feels the need to interfere in our life, we must see it for what it is, and that it is just their opinion. It is not our truth and it is only us that knows our own truth.

When the opinions of others have caused us doubt, we can close our eyes, and ask our heart what we need to know. Our heart knows more than anyone else what is best for us. Our heart knows more than our minds what our purpose is. Our heart through the soul holds the link to our higher self, and it will speak if we listen.

To listen, we must close off the sound of others and not overthink with our minds. Our heart cannot communicate with us in the noise of others and the noise of our minds. When we clear the internal noise of our minds, and the external noise of others, the heart will speak.

When we listen to our heart, we can hear our own truth. Once we know our truth, we can know the way to live our purpose and fulfil our dreams. When we know our own heart, we know who we are, and we know how to live our life as we are meant to. When we know our own heart, we need not let the opinions or actions of others move us from our centre. We need not let others decide for us as it is through the heart, we will find our way, our path and our truth.

CHAPTER 6

HEALTH: STOP STRESS

When faced with trauma, or bad news, our physical bodies go into an automatic stress response. This response is our inbuilt alarm system, designed to pump our body full of adrenaline. This adrenaline provides us with the additional physical energy needed to fight or flight the perceived threat that has jeopardised our safety.

In a normal stress response, and once the threat is over, the body returns to its natural state of balance. Unfortunately, there are times when the stress response does not switch off and remains running. When this happens, it will continue to erode the body of its energy and vitality. Over time, the depletion will negatively affect the physical body.

The long-term effects of ongoing stress on the body cannot be underestimated. Stress interferes and impacts the balance of our nervous and lymphatic systems. The normal functioning of these systems is vital for our long-term health and wellbeing. Once these systems are out of balance, the organs to which they support are impacted.

The impacts of stress on the body is a major contributory factor to many diseases and can also be the final straw that will bring a disease to the fore. When diagnosed with a disease, the diagnosis itself can bring on additional emotional stress and slow down the chances we have of healing from the disease.

Stress on top of more stress continues to deplete the body of the vital energy needed to naturally heal the body. Stress impacts our stomach, heart, nervous system, sleep, and appetite, which are all essential towards our natural healing. It is ironic that at a time of us needing to heal the most, it can be blocked by the very emotional stress of having and living with a disease.

The emotional stress of a diagnosis is compounded by the additional financial stress. The diagnosis might result in us no longer being able to work and financially support ourselves. It is also a time of expensive medical bills. We can find ourselves overwhelmed by stress.

There is no easy way to deal with stress during these times. We can only take each day as it comes and not look too far into the future. We can try to lower our stress through gentle exercise, talking to a loved one, and choosing positive thoughts where possible.

It is only in reducing our stress that we can give our bodies the best chance towards healing. It is only in overcoming the stress that we may begin to see the light at the end of the tunnel. It is only in releasing stress that we can allow our true power to come through. Our true ability to heal and our ability to cope, even in the darkest situations.

WEALTH: HELP OTHERS

When we think of others less fortunate than us, we can gain some perspective on practicing gratitude. When we think about those who lay lonely in hospital beds, those who cannot afford to eat or those who have lost a loved one, we can start to shift to a place of gratitude in our own life. We can start to shift to a place of wanting to help others.

When we shift our thinking towards others in need, we shift our energy from self to the collective. By moving our mind from self to the needs of others, we can move away from our own feelings of loneliness. We can gain a new perspective on our own life by helping others. In helping others, we can help ourselves.

There is always someone in need of a helping hand. A lonely neighbour, an elderly relative or someone living on the streets can be helped by simply giving them our time. As a result of unfortunate life circumstance, those without a home or without a family need our help in whatever way we can afford to give it. Those who are lonely, need our time in whatever way we can spare it.

When we do give, we should give freely and not have expectations for getting anything back in return. We should not give to gain recognition and praise from others. This is self-interested giving. We should give from a place of genuinely wanting to help someone else in need. We should give from a place of compassion. A place from the heart.

When we give from the heart and give freely without expectation, the feeling of giving to another is more rewarding than holding possession of the material thing that is given. Giving, never takes away from what we have, as it will flow back to us. It flows freely back to us when we give freely and from a genuine place.

As a collective, we are all connected by energy. This energy, not visible to the naked eye flows between us and through us. We exchange this energy to one another, both positive and negative. When we participate in the act of helping each other, we allow the positive energy flow from us and therefore it flows back to us. When we act selfishly, we cut off that energy flow so eventually those who do not give, end up losing that in which they held on to. By holding, they have blocked themselves from the collective and blocked themselves from receiving.

We should try to spread our love as far and as wide as we can. We can give little too many and not a lot to a few. We should not only give to our loved ones. We should give what we have to charity and strangers. We can spread what we have to as many as we can, always focusing on those most in need of our help. If we had nothing else to give but our time to those around us who are lonely then we would be giving the most powerful thing of all, and that is our love.

HAPPINESS: GRATITUDE II

Even in our darkest hour, or most stressful day, there is always something to be grateful for. Whether it is the roof over our head, the food in our fridge or the clothes on our back, we must remind ourselves that we are privileged. We must remember that there are many in our world who go without these basic needs. The gift of simply being alive is a privilege. If we can think of nothing else, we can be grateful for our breath.

We live in a society of consumerism, always wanting more and always comparing what we have to that of others. We live in a society of demand. Two clicks and two days later and we can have what we want to arrive at our front door. In the middle of all the consuming, we never stop to think that we might have enough. We never stop to find gratitude in what we do have.

It is easy to find gratitude in our everyday lives. From the moment we wake up, we can give thanks for our bed, sleep, and warmth. We can give thanks for our first ;;breath and for the gift of movement. When we can freely move and get out of bed, we can find gratitude. When we get out of bed with a grateful attitude, it will have a positive impact on the rest of our day.

We can take so much of our lives for granted and it is usually for the simple things. It is easy to become complacent for all that we have, and we begin to expect it to be that way. We expect it and then we expect more. We look at what we do not have and we long for it. We convince ourselves, that when we have this or that, we will finally be happy.

When we are in a state of wanting or longing, we are in a state of future happiness. Our happiness is always dependent on something that has not yet happened. It is dependent on something that might not happen. When we are in this state, we can never really experience happiness in the present moment, and we can never really experience life as it is.

When we choose to express our life from a place of gratitude and abundance, we will start to realise how wealthy we really are. We will start to see our wealth, in the simple things and the simple life. From this place of gratitude, we will attract more and more reasons into our life to be grateful. From this place, our happiness stays in the now.

When we ask for something from a place within our heart and our intentions are good, then if meant for us, it will eventually find its way to us. When we ask sincerely and with gratitude, we increase our chances to receive what it is we are seeking. When we find the gratitude for the simple things in life, we will start to enjoy life in its simplicity. We will start to enjoy life from a place in our heart, a place of thanks, and a place of happiness.

LOVE: BE YOUR OWN REASON

Whatever we choose as our reason for change, our primary reason should be for ourselves. We should always be our own reason. Our reason to change, our reason to love and our reason to forgive. We should never change because somebody else has told us to or because we want acceptance from another. It must come from within, the decision and the power to change.

All change is difficult, and we will face numerous obstacles along the way. We will face failure and we will face challenges. We will be tested over and over again, and we must learn how to persist and hold the belief that we can and we will. We must build our resilience and keep the faith at the times when it seems easier to give up. By committing to change, we commit to ourselves.

In getting through the change, whatever this may be, we must continually remind ourselves of our own reason. We must remember the why. We must remember our decision. If our reason was for someone else, it will be difficult to reach our goal, and it will be difficult to stay motivated. It will be difficult to see it through if we were not our own reason.

We should always remember that we are worth the change and we are worth the fight. We are worth the good health, the good life and we deserve all the good that life has to offer. We must start each day and take on the fight for ourselves. The fight to change, and the fight to be well.

We must be ready to fight our own battles as there is no one else that can take them on for us. We can rest and we can take a break, but we must never give up on ourselves. We must never let go of the hope. The hope that anything and everything is possible. The hope that we can achieve our dreams and that we deserve them.

When we become our own reason for all that we do in life, we shift to a place of self-love and self-belief. From this place, we can find our inner resilience and perseverance to see our dreams through even in the days that we are tested. From this place, we can tap into a place of inner strength and determination. From this place, we can stay on our path and remain true to ourselves.

When we become our own reason for all that we do in life and fulfil our own basic needs then we can help others from a place of abundance. If we have not met our own basic needs first, we can become easily drained or resentful in helping others.

When we choose to be our own reason and put our own basic needs first, we act in self-love. When we love ourselves, we can love others. When we help ourselves, we can help others. In being our own reason, we stay true to who we are and what we want in life. We stay true to our heart and grow from a place of love. From this place we can share our love freely with others.

CHAPTER 7

HEALTH: THERE IS
NO MAGIC PILL*

When disease presents in the body, there is seldom just one cause or reason for it for it. It is caused by a cumulation of underlying factors from our inner and outer environments. The cause is interconnected to several factors such as genes, physical exercise, diet, our emotional state and stress levels. As the cause is cumulative, the cure is also cumulative.

Healing for any disease can only be achieved by having an open mind and a holistic view of health. Each contributory factor needs assessment. Often, when we seek a medical opinion, the primary focus is towards medication or surgery. It is therefore up to us to look at the full picture for full health. We must acknowledge each underlying factor that exists and make the necessary lifestyle changes for each.

Medication alone, although necessary, is not the only solution in achieving long term wellness and health. Medication cannot cure a disease. Medication can only minimize the effect of the disease on the body. It can buy us time and it can reduce the symptoms of the disease, but it will not cure the body of the disease. The disease continues to exist alongside the medication.

As the disease continues to exist, the dependency and reliance on the medication will also continue to exist. It is often necessary to increase the dosage to maintain the same effects over time. Medication comes with its very own side effects and we can soon find ourselves in a vicious cycle of needing more and more medication to keep covering up each symptom.

Medication can play a part as a short-term solution while we establish a longer-term plan for wellness. Medication can be used effectively while we make longer term positive lifestyle changes to address the underlying causes of our disease. If we rely solely on medication as the solution for our healing, we can never fully address the underlying factors towards long term health. Unfortunately, there is no such thing as a magic pill when it comes to our health.

When we look at the full picture for health, we give ourselves the best chance for healing and reducing the impacts of living with a disease. There are always multiple factors at play when it comes to addressing our health and by opening our minds to all the options available to us, we open ourselves to all the possibilities for healing.

Our healing and long-term health is unique and personal to each one of us. It is a journey we must all face at some time or another and it is only by taking the journey that we can know what is right for us and what works for us. It is only on our journey that we will find our own path towards health and healing, in whatever form that may take, we must always take faith and hope with us.

*It is important to seek and consult with medical advice before reducing, or stopping any medication prescribed.

WEALTH: KNOW YOUR OWN PASSION

Each day is a new opportunity to learn and to grow. No matter what age we become, we should never stop learning, or following our passion. We must always be willing to pursue our dream in life. We deserve to learn and live through our passion. We deserve to find happiness in our work.

When we were younger, learning may have been a negative experience for us. We may have studied subjects that we had no interest in. Regardless of this experience, we hold the power today to choose what it is we want to learn. We can choose to learn from a place of passion instead of obligation.

If we can find our passion is and create a career from it, we can find true happiness. If we enjoy what we do, it never has to seem like work. If we are working through our passion, it never has to feel like we are draining our energy from work. When it is our passion, we gain energy from it instead.

It is easy to fall into a career path driven by the desire and need for money. The more money we make, the more we fall into the trap of working to financially maintain a certain lifestyle. Before we choose our career path, we should stop and think of the price we will pay in exchange for the financial reward. When we choose work that is not aligned to our passion, we drain ourselves of our energy and this will soon start to impact other aspects of our life.

It can be better to live with less and to enjoy what we do. If we enjoy our work and are passionate about it, we can be successful at it, and over time the finances will flow to us. It may take time and it may take patience but the emotional reward for doing what we love will always outweigh the initial lack of having financial resources.

When we discover our true passion and work at what we love to do, we become full of enthusiasm and positive energy which is infectious to other people. We can attract success from this energy. We can attract the right people into our lives to help us to succeed with this energy.

It may take time for us to discover our passion. A career choice may not always work out and we may have to stick with it for a time because of personal commitments and obligation. During these times, it may be difficult to see the way out and our only option is to wait and put our passion on hold.

When we are ready, and the timing is right, it is never too late for us to choose what it is we want to learn and to start over. Our lives are short, and our work will be our legacy. It will become what gets left behind. It is through our work that we can share our true skills and live our true-life purpose. It is only us that can know our passion. It is only us that can choose our path. Our path is our passion.

HAPPINESS: REMOVE JUDGEMENT

Judgement is everywhere and judgement is within all of us. Without even being aware, we spend significant amounts of time judging one another and judging ourselves. Our outer judgement is generally a reflection of our inner judgement. We all have insecurities, and we may deal with these by projecting them back on to the world in the form of judgement.

We are taught not to judge a book by its cover, but this is exactly what we all do. We are guilty of judging at face value and judging on outer appearance. We judge without ever really knowing a person, a situation or what someone else is going through. We judge others to temporarily make ourselves feel better. We judge to create our own outer superiority. We judge to mask our own inner inferiority.

We are quick to judge a person's physical appearance or what they own. If they have too much, we judge them and if they have too little, we judge them too. If they are overweight or too thin, we are judging. Even when we see somebody with the perfect body, we find a reason to judge. Sadly, there is always a reason for judgement.

There is no one that is protected from our judgement. We judge our closest family, strangers, and close friends. Regardless of whether we know someone or not, we can judge them. We are so busy judging on the outside that we do not stop to think where all the judgement is coming from. We do not question where the inferiority complex is coming from. We do not question why we need to compare. We do not question whether we could feel good without judgement.

We all know on some level that there is nothing to gain in judging one other. There is no reason to feel inferior of another because they have more. Equally, there is no reason to feel superior of another because they have less. Why does it really matter what we own? Why does it really matter to compare? What are we gaining from our judgments?

There is nothing to gain by looking for a reason to judge. If we look at our inner judgement, we might start to realise the reasons for our outer judgement. Our judgement is only ever a reflection of what is going on inside. When we address the inner, we can remove the outer.

The differences between how we look or what we own need not be a reason for judgement. In judgement, we create a reason to feel resentment and jealousy towards each other. When we look at the real reason that we judge and remove it, we can begin to accept others and come together despite our differences. We can become united in understanding each other without judgement.

LOVE: PLANET EARTH

We can find many reasons to love our world when we sit in nature. We can find love by the water, among the trees and with animals. We can find love spending time at the sea with the sand on our feet and the air on our faces. Our planet earth gives us much to love and be thankful for.

Our planet earth knows nothing but giving. It gives us the air that we breathe, the food that we eat, the water that we drink and the light that we need. It has given us the perfect cycles, of seasons, of time, of light and of dark. It is perfect in every sense and needs no input from us to operate. It needs no interference from us to be.

Unfortunately for the planet, we do interfere, and we interfere in a negative way. We cut our trees, we pollute our waters, the land and our sky's and we continue to take what we want with no end in sight. We take from it as if it is an endless commodity. We take in greed and we take with no thought for the future of mankind.

There is nothing on earth or in life that can sustain such taking. It goes against all the laws, that we can take without consequence and that we can take without losing it all. Planet earth is no different and it cannot and will not sustain all the taking. It has come a time for us to give back, and to stop all the taking. It has come a time for us to open our eyes and to save what we have left.

We can all play a part in giving back and in the collective effort to love our planet. We can all make the effort to plant and grow trees and to care for animals. We can all reduce our waste and pollution. We can all make a difference to protect and save our planet.

We may be slow to act because we believe that we are not directly impacted by climate change or that it does not exist. The truth is that our climate has changed and the most vulnerable are paying the price. If we opened are eyes to it, we could reduce the impact and slow down the change.

We may be slow to act because we believe we cannot make any difference. By doing nothing, we are making excuses for an inconvenient truth. Individually, we hold the power to do good things. Collectively, we hold the power to do great things. We can look to a young girl from Sweden to see the impact of one individual. To see the power of one young individual with a voice.

We are living on a planet that has become a ticking time bomb because of our interference and it is only a matter of time before we will see the real consequences unfold. We cannot afford to wait anymore. We cannot afford to make excuses anymore. Like the young girl from Sweden, we must find our voice, and we must stand up for what is right. We must stand up for planet earth. We must stand up and be counted for our future. For the future of others and for the future of mankind.

CHAPTER 8

HEALTH: PREPARE FOR THE EXPECTED

When we save for the rainy day, we can be prepared for the difficult times that lie ahead. In these times we will need physical, mental and financial reserves in place. We will need extra fat to burn. If we are depleted at these times, the road back is longer and harder. If we have maintained our health as best as we can in the good times, we can face the harder times stronger.

In preparing for these times, we prepare for the expected. We will all have challenges to face at some time or another. When we have our reserves in place, we can overcome what we need to as best we can. We give ourselves the best chance of survival. We give ourselves the best chance to fight.

We can choose to be active instead of reactive in preparing to cope for these times. We can focus our energy into maintaining ourselves as best as we can in the good times. We can focus our attention on setting aside our reserves and building our resilience. We can reduce our mental stress knowing that we have reserves in place when we need them.

When we have financial reserves in place, we can have peace of mind. If we need to take time off to rest, we can do so without the stress of worrying how we pay bills. Our reserves will help us to pay for the help that we might need from others. Our financial reserves give us the freedom of choice and the freedom from additional financial stress.

When we reduce our mental stress during difficult times, we can improve our ability to cope and to think clearly. In stressful situations, our mind can be our own worst enemy for imagining a worst-case scenario. At these times, we must remain mindful and bring our thoughts back using positive affirmations and beliefs. We must remind ourselves that we are stronger than we think and more resilient then we know.

We can be active in improving our immune system to help us to physically heal during difficult times. It can be boosted by diet, exercise and meditation. Our bodies are designed to cope and heal from many foreign bodies. We can facilitate our healing ability in advance by building our immune system and keeping it as strong as it can be.

When we direct our energy into what we can prepare for, we focus on the positive. If we direct our energy into worry and stress, we reduce our ability to build our reserves and we weaken our immune system. In preparation, we choose a position of power over a position of defeat. We choose to build our reserves as best as we can when we can. We choose to be active instead of reactive in preparing for the expected.

WEALTH: GETTING OUT OF OUR WAY

By being stubborn, we stand in our own way. When we feel that we know best and are always right, we stand in our own way. This feeling blocks us from the knowledge and guidance of others and holds us back in life. To move forward in life, we must literally get out of our own way. To move forward with others, we must remain open to others, and open to the collective learning from others.

Knowing who we are and being confident in our own decision making is important, but it is also important to seek the guidance and advice of others in certain situations. By admitting that we do not always know the answer and acknowledging that someone else might know better, we open ourselves up to the collective and let go of our own ego.

Admitting when we are wrong and learning from our mistakes takes enormous courage. We are inclined to protect our own ego so it can be difficult to admit when we make a mistake. It can be difficult to admit that another knows best. It can speak more of a person's character when they are open to taking on another's, advice and to admit when they were wrong. It takes courage to say; "the advice you gave me really helped and I am glad I listened, thank you for giving it to me".

Staying open and accepting what someone else has to say, especially if it differs from our own point of view can help us build our personal relationships and our tolerance towards others. It can help us build our own character. In accepting another viewpoint, we need not change ours, but in acceptance comes understanding and in understanding comes growth. If we remain open to each other, we might learn something new. By being open, we can always receive something new.

There are some that will never be able to get out of their own way. They will remain stuck in old habits and beliefs. They will remain stuck in their opinions. The more time we practice being open minded, the more we can identify with others who are also open minded. When we choose to become aware, we choose our company wisely and we choose how we use our energy wisely. When we begin to change ourselves, we change those who are around us. We change the energy that we attract.

In getting out of our own way, we begin to let go of our need to be right, and our need to protect our ego. By protecting this need, we are held back. By distancing ourselves from our ego, we free ourselves of the need to be right. When we free ourselves, we allow life to flow freely before us and around us. We allow others to play a part, we play a part in the collective, and we play a part in life. When we get out of our own way, we begin to see the way. The way of our light, and the way with others.

HAPPINESS: LIMIT THE NEGATIVE

The negative is all around us. It is on the news, the radio, social media, and it is within all of us. Once we become consciously aware of negative sources, we can choose to limit our time listening or paying attention to it. We can aim to reduce our intake over time to zero tolerance and acceptance.

It is never too late to start to choose each day our thoughts and our company. It is never too late to decide what situations no longer serve us. It is never too late to walk away. We always have a choice when it comes to protecting our mental health. We should choose what feels right for us, as we will never keep everyone happy. It is not our job to keep everyone happy.

We may not be able to go from one hundred to zero overnight, and it may take us a lifetime to shift our world to a place of positive people and places. The important thing is, that we start. That we start becoming aware of the negative noise around us and that we start choosing the positive where possible. Over time our small choices towards the positive, will add up.

When it is not possible to walk away from a negative situation, we must look at protecting ourselves in other ways. We must become aware of protecting our energy and not get drawn into the drama of other people. There will be some that will always want drama in their life. We must place our boundaries firmly in place. We must be selfish in the pursuit of the positive.

We can start by taking a check of where and when we are absorbing negative news and people. Once we become aware of where our energy is being drained, we can start to make some positive decisions. We can decide what to remove immediately and what might need to be phased out over time. With practice and awareness, we will become much better at removing ourselves from negative situations as soon as they appear in our lives. We will stop making excuses for them to stick around.

When we listen to the negative, we absorb the negative. It becomes a negative energy that our mind and body will either process or store. This energy is either processed and released or stored somewhere in the mind or body. When we limit our intake of the negative, we reduce the negative load for the body to process or store.

When those around us are speaking negatively, we can practice the act of disengagement from them. We can disengage from them by not participating in what they are saying. We can consciously hand it back to them to process while we can stay grounded in the positive. We can choose not to participate mentally or emotionally in their negativity. We can choose to remain in our own positive power. We can choose to say no. No to the negative.

LOVE: IN FRIENDSHIP

Our friends come in all shapes and sizes. Each friendship will bring a different dynamic into our life and a different teaching and experience. Each friendship is unique, and some can last the test of time and distance, while others will not. Sometimes we need to let go of a friendship and know that it has come to an end. We can let it go in love and in gratitude.

We can feel disappointed when our friends respond differently to how we would respond to them. When we hold expectations for how they should respond to us, we set them up to fail and we set ourselves up for disappointment. When we expect our friends to change for us, we create ongoing feelings of resentment and conflict in the relationship.

We cannot expect our friends to respond or to change as we would because of our unique life experiences and differences. When we accept our differences, we avoid unnecessary conflict and disappointment. Sometimes the differences will be so far apart that a relationship will dissolve. Sometimes the difference can bring growth, acceptance, understanding and teaching into our lives.

Knowing a friend for who they are and not who we expect them to be can save us from suffering. Knowing and accepting each other at face value allows us to decide where we fit into our life and them to ours. Sometimes there is no place. Sometimes we are just meant to have brief encounters.

Like love, each friendship is a friendship worth having even if it is temporary. Each friendship will hold a unique place in our heart and in our memories. Each one will store the memories that can remind us how to laugh, and how to remember the good times. Our memories can remind us of the lighter times and when life was not so complicated.

We can reach out to an old friend and feel that no time has passed between us at all. An old friendship can be reignited and come back into our lives in the most unexpected way. It can come back with more meaning and appreciation than before. It can grow into a different type of friendship than before. A true friendship will find its way back to us, regardless of time or distance.

Whether it is a new or an old friendship, a true friendship accepts and values all that a person is. It includes love and forgiveness, laughter and tears, growth, and support of each other. Our friends become the teachers and the family we get to choose.

When we know each other for who we are, we understand each other. When we understand each other, we can grow in love together. We can use our differences as a reason to learn acceptance and patience instead of a reason for conflict and hate. When we accept each other for who we are, we can come together in love regardless of where we have come from or where we are going. In friendship, we can learn to love in difference.

CHAPTER 9

HEALTH: CONSTANT COMPLAINING

We will find that once we consciously begin to choose a positive path in our life, that negative thoughts will stop coming, and that those around us respect our new positive outlook. There will always be times when negative influences are unavoidable but if they are limited, they will limit their effect on our health. The more time and effort we spend in positive company, the more positive our minds will become.

When someone is constantly complaining around us, they drain us of our life energy. When someone is constantly complaining, we must create awareness and detachment from it to protect our mental health. Through awareness, we can detach from their personal discontentment and preserve our positive energy. We can preserve our good health.

When we complain, we choose the negative and offload onto someone else, instead of taking our own personal responsibility for what it is we need to change. We create a situation where we get to play a victim, yet we hold our own free will to change the very thing we choose to complain about.

Complaining reduces our ability to offer gratitude for all that life has to offer us. When we complain, we move to a position of finding something wrong instead of choosing something that is right. If we keep choosing all that is right, we will start to see all that is right in ourselves and in others too. In choosing all that is right, we choose to have a positive mind and positive health.

When we stop and become aware of how much complaining goes on around us, we may be surprised. It is everywhere. It is in our families, among our friends and on the news. It is near impossible to go a day without witnessing someone else complaining

When we start to reduce our complaining, we will begin to improve our mental health. When we become aware of it, we can change the pattern and we can choose the opposite, a compliment. When there is no compliment to give, then we need say nothing at all.

In reducing our habit of complaining, we will begin to realise that we are all trying our best in life for ourselves and for each other. In recognising all that is good in each other, we can stop living in a world of expected perfection.

The expectation for perfection gives us a reason to complain. The acceptance of imperfection gives us a reason to offer gratitude. It gives us a reason to accept each other and accept ourselves. It gives us a reason to love, love in the flow of life, love in the flow of change, and love in imperfection.

WEALTH: A JOURNEY OF SELF BELIEF

Self-belief is an output of self-love. One cannot exist without the other. When we believe that we can, and that we will, we can achieve anything that our mind can imagine. Knowing that we can is much more powerful then knowing how we will. We do not always need a concrete plan. We do not need to know the exact path, just the general direction in which we are going and the belief to back ourselves along the way.

When we have chosen our path and the direction of our journey, we will face many bumps along the road. We will face many decisions that will change our direction. There will be times when we face a mountain and other times a peaceful lake. As we walk through life, we are best to surround ourselves with those who share our belief that even if it takes time, we can climb any mountain.

When we begin to climb our mountain, we are best to let go of those who are stuck at the bottom. We are best to continue without them and allow them to start their own journey in their own time. Sometimes we cannot afford to wait for them, and our journey takes a different path. We must continue on our own path, trusting that when the timing is right, we will meet again.

When we have self-belief and surround ourselves with those who believe in us, we will be consistent and resilient on our journey. We will know that there will be days when we do not move forward and days when we go backwards. Our self-belief will be the reason that we start each new day in hope. Hope to try again and pick ourselves up again.

As we continue our journey, we must remember and acknowledge how far we have come and not how far we have left to go. We must remember to stop, breath and take in the beauty that surrounds us. We must remember that it is ok to take a break and to rest.

Our journey gives us an opportunity to offer gratitude and love with those who have shared it with us. By standing together, we have stood stronger than if we had gone it alone. Together we have kept the hope alive in achieving our goal. Together we have faced and overcome defeat.

Step by step, little by little, day by day, our efforts will soon add up and be rewarded. When we keep the faith, the belief and the determination inside that anything is possible, we can stay on the road even when the journey seems long, and we get tired.

How we navigate our journey in life is in our hands. We can choose the pace and the people that will join us. We can choose to take in each moment. We can choose to be present along our way. We can choose to believe. By believing in ourselves, we can believe in each other, and we can believe in the possibilities of our journey together and the possibilities of our life.

HAPPINESS: THE TRUTH LIES WITHIN

We always know the answer we are looking for, but sometimes we are not ready to hear our own truth. Our infinite intelligence holds the truth that we are looking for but often we can look towards others to answer our truth for us. Fortunately for us, it is only us that know our own truth.

When the timing is right and we are ready, we will hear the truth we need to make our decisions and move forward in our lives. Often, because of fear, it is easier to hide away from our truth, and hide away from the world. It is easier to ignore our truth.

Sometimes the answer we are looking for is standing right in front of us and it will remain there, waiting for us until we are ready to listen. It may take a lifetime for us to be ready to hear our own truth. To hear it, we need to be in the right space to receive it, both mentally and emotionally.

When we are ready to listen, we might be surprised that we had not listened to it earlier but there is nothing to gain in regret. We can be proud that we have started to listen. We have taken the first step. We are honouring ourselves with our own truth. We can move forward in positive self-belief and encouragement instead of critical regret.

Sometimes we may have to wait patiently for those that we love to face their own truth. It may seem obvious to us, but we must respect that they will receive it but only when they are ready. As we wait, we can support them with patience and love. As we wait, we can support them with the space they need in facing their truth.

We can encourage a loved one to face their own truth, but we can never place our own expectations on when they will receive it. We can never live another's life for them. We can never live their truth for them. We can only speak and live our own truth and live our own life.

Timing and circumstance are needed to hear our own truth. When they align, magic things can happen. Sometimes our truth comes when we are least expecting it. Other times, we must be patient until it does. As we wait, we can close our eyes and take a deep breath to come into the present moment. From here, we can tap into our inner voice. We can ask ourselves our very own questions and if we are open to it, we will hear the answers.

Our truth does not come from the mind. It does not come from the logical, or the rational. When we find the answers within and offer gratitude, we can deepen our connection to this place of inner truth. When we begin to trust this source, we may never have to question ourselves again. Our truth will flow freely and guide us on our path. It will guide us in love. It will guide us home.

LOVE: A HIGHER POWER

No matter what form it takes, we are all free to believe in a higher spiritual power. This power may be called God, Source or the Divine. Sometimes the form may be nothing at all. Our spiritual beliefs are unique to each of us and they vary across every religion, country, and race.

In whatever form we have decided our belief to be, our free choice and decision deserves respect from others. Our spiritual choices and beliefs are personal to each of us and may change several times during our lifetime. Sometimes, we may have multiple and interchangeable beliefs.

Developing a belief in a higher power can enhance our lives. It can give us a deeper purpose and meaning to life and how we live it. Our beliefs can provide us with comfort and guidance when we need it the most. Our beliefs can direct us on the right path and surround us with the energy and courage to continue when our human strength is tested.

When we find and develop spiritual beliefs, they become our sacred space for peace and healing. That will be the place we will go to find the answers. That will be the place we will go to remember a loved one and to remember how to love ourselves.

Our different beliefs need not be a reason for debate or conflict. A higher power may be communicating to us in several forms and each of us picks up this communication on a different level. We all relate to it differently. It will have a specific and unique meaning to each of us, based on our individual life circumstances and experiences.

Sometimes we choose to pray to a higher power and perform specific rituals based on our beliefs. It is fascinating to explore the different ways in which this is done across the world. If we open our mind to it, we may experience something special or something new from the belief of others. A new experience might lead us on a different path and journey. It may provide us with some form of healing.

A higher belief at its core is always based on love. It has been created for us in love and we are all held in this love until we return. A higher power has created us all equal. A higher power has given us the free will and choice to hold our own beliefs. If we are given this free will from above, then it must be respected below.

If our beliefs are a reason for conflict, we are all equally responsible to pursue peace regardless of our chosen beliefs. We are all equally responsible to respect each other for the time that we have left. Our beliefs are never a reason for conflict, or a reason to hate. Our beliefs are a reason to love, and a reason to respect.

CHAPTER 10

HEALTH: GOING AGAINST YOUR GUT

We have two types of intelligence available to us. There is mental intelligence and there is gut intelligence. The later by-passes the mind. It knows the answer without having to consult the mind. The answer is based on a feeling inside. A gut feeling.

Bypassing our gut feeling and ignoring it will often result in us making the wrong decision or taking the wrong path. We may end up staying in a situation that we are not happy in. We may end up living through a situation that no longer serves us. We may end up accepting less than our hearts desire.

A gut feeling is our sixth sense. It comes from a place that we cannot rationalise. It comes from a place of feeling. It does not come from a place of ration or reason. It comes from our connection to a higher source. It is our infinite intelligence.

Many successful people have tuned into this intelligence to make the decisions that have brought them their success. They have trusted that the information they need is already at hand. They trust the information despite logic. They trust their gut feeling and are usually right, even against the odds.

It is only by listening and trusting our gut feeling that we improve our communication with it. It is only by quieting the mind that we can hear it. We can quieten the mind by meditation or exercise. When we are in this state, the answer will speak. The answer will come.

An animal has developed this sixth sense for their survival. They sense danger when it is near. The danger is not always visible, but they feel it and they act on that feeling and flee. They do not wait around, questioning it. They accept their infinite intelligence at face value. They use it to survive.

As humans, we have created a degree of separation from it. We overthink, over analyse, and are influenced by what others have to say. When we feel our sixth sense, we can ignore it, and use excuses as to why we have not listened. We try to rationalise it and choose the decision of the mind. We question it and choose the decision of others.

Sometimes we know what we know, and we do not know how we know. That is our sixth sense. When it arises again, welcome it, thank it, and it will return stronger and better. Once we re-establish our connection to it, it will bring us on the right path time and time again. It will bring us success time and time again. It will redirect our journey time and time again. Our journey of love. Our journey home.

WEALTH: THE LIGHTER SIDE

We all feel lighter after a good laugh. We all feel better when we see someone else smile. When things become heavy, we can try to lighten the load and see the lighter side of life. It does not always have to be so serious. We do not have to be so serious.

As we grow up, we physically outgrow our physical child, but our inner child remains. She never leaves us. She waits for us to have fun again. She waits for us to get on the trampoline again. She is ready for us to let go and be free again.

We are never too old to play, despite how old we have become. Our problems can melt away in the presence of play and in laughter. Our problems can temporarily disappear when we let our inner child out to play.

When we play, we can see the lighter side of life, even in a difficult situation. We can see the light at the end of the tunnel. When we remember a good childhood memory, we can remember how it felt when life was fun, and life was lighter.

When we go back to what life was like in our early years, we can remember a simpler life. We can remember how it felt to play and to laugh. We can remember how it felt not to be afraid. We might have to grow old, but we stay young at heart when we connect to our inner child. We are never too old to play and we will never grow old in laughter.

When we have a sense of humour and learn how to laugh at ourselves, it might help us lighten a difficult situation. It might help us to see the good side of life and remind us of the lighter side again. It may even give us some perspective of our situation and turn it around on its head.

When we laugh, we get the physical benefits for the body as we release tension and hormones that help us to deal with stress. When we laugh, we get the mental benefits as we are taken into the present moment and in that moment, we can forget our troubles and in our worries.

When we make time for having fun, we make time to stay young. Even though we have grown old and have responsibility, we can live our lives on the lighter side. When we inject a sense of fun into our lives and relationships, we stay young in our minds and hearts.

When we laugh, we live in the present, we love in the present and we connect to our beautiful inner child in the present. When we play, we connect to our beautiful self and even if for a moment, we are transported to that part of life that is good again and that part of life that is worth living. Living lighter and living in laughter.

HAPPINESS: KNOW YOUR OWN BUSINESS

In our hearts we have good intentions for each other, and we want the best for each other. Although our intentions are good, it can also mean that we are involved in each other's business and we are involved in each other's lives. We create crossed boundaries when we take on the business of another.

Boundaries can be crossed within families and with close friends. In these relationships, we might feel it is our business as to what decisions are made. The truth is, it is none of our business and it is only them that will live with the consequence.

Unless there is a direct consequence for us, then it is none of our business. If it does not directly impact us financially, physically, or mentally, then it is none of our business. If it is none of our business, we must walk away. We must let it be and turn our attention to our own business.

We may think that we know what is best for a loved one, but we can only ever know what is best for ourselves. It is easy to hide away behind the perceived responsibility of others. It is easy to hide away from our own life. It is easy to hide away by trying to own the life of others or decide the life of others.

We can only offer support from the side-lines for our loved ones. We cannot decide for them. We cannot live their life for them. We must respect them, their journey, and their chosen path even if it differs from what we had hoped and what we think is right.

We can offer advice if we are asked. If not, then it is none of our business. If we are giving opinions when it is none of our business, we are wasting our time and our energy when it is needed in sorting our own business.

There will be times when our loved ones do not need our help and they do not need us. They do not need to hear what we have to say, and they need their own time and space. The space between us is not a reason to stop loving them and we can continue to support them from a distance. We can be patient and ready for them when they do ask for our help.

When we remove our attention from the lives of others, we can move the focus towards our own lives. When we remove ourselves from the business of others, we will have healthier relationships with those around us and with ourselves.

We will be surprised how much time we can free up in our own lives once we identify what is and not our business. We will be amazed at what we can achieve by putting our energy and attention into ourselves over others. We can still love and support each other with space and distance in between. We can still share our journey among the boundaries.

LOVE: SELF WORTH

The easiest way to start having what we really want is to start with the belief that we are worth it and fully deserve it. We can build on this belief by opening our hearts to receiving it and once we receive it, we can offer gratitude for it. This becomes the cycle of abundance. The cycle of holding the belief, remaining open to receiving it, and offering gratitude when it comes.

Self-worth is an output of self-belief. The belief comes from a feeling deep within that we deserve having what we want. The belief is a feeling that we deserve the best in life. It is knowing that we deserve the best from our relationships and the best from our home and work environments.

Self-worth is a belief that we do not settle for any less than we are worth. It is a belief that we speak up when our standards are comprised or when our boundaries are crossed. It is finding our voice and not being afraid of what other people think. It is not changing because of what other people say.

When we were young, we were taught not to be greedy and to be happy with what we have. This teaching leads us to expect little from what life has to offer and it teaches us to settle. There is a difference in knowing our self-worth and being selfish or self-centred. When our self-worth comes from our heart, it is pure, and we will equally want the best for others. Our self-worth is not motivated by greed, as it is motivated in love.

When we know that we deserve the absolute best out of life, this will be reflected in the relationships that we have with ourselves and with others. It will reflect how we expect to be treated and respected by others and it will reflect our ability to walk away when a situation no longer serves us. It will mirror our ability and resilience to seek what it is, we are looking for.

When we believe there is not enough to go around for everyone, we can act out in greed. When we act in greed, we act in self and remove our ability to share our wealth with others. When we act in greed, we cut ourselves from the collective and from receiving.

The power lies within us to change our circumstances by removing our limiting beliefs and replacing them with new unlimiting beliefs of abundance through receiving and giving. We all hold the power to start telling ourselves a different story and to manifest what it is we believe we deserve.

There is no difference between each of us and our ability in achieving our dreams. The only difference that separates us is the belief that we hold of our self-worth. This belief with either block or facilitate us in achieving our success in life. This belief will manifest in us receiving what it is we truly desire. In knowing our self-worth, we know that we are worth all the good that life has to offer us, and we will want the same for others.

CHAPTER 11

HEALTH: THE POWER OF SURRENDER

We carry much around from day to day. We carry much of ourselves and of others. We carry it all in our heads. We can be consumed with worry as we are caught up anticipating the future or held back by fear of the past. We can become stuck in our lives and in our worries.

We move away from living in the present when we allow the actions of the past or the untold future hold us in a state that is neither past nor present. This state blocks us from life, it blocks us from our energy, and it can become heavy as we struggle to release the old or feel overcome by the new.

The past does not dictate our future and our future does not dictate the present. The only thing we can be sure of is today and the moment before us. We can free ourselves from the actions of the past or what may happen in the future when we come into the present moment.

When we feel overwhelmed by life or when life becomes heavy, we can take a moment to pause, to slow down and to breath. We can take a moment to surrender. We can surrender our worries, our fears, and our anxieties. We can surrender to a higher power.

Our minds can become lighter when we surrender our worries. We can surrender and trust that we are held and supported by a higher power. When we feel supported, we may find strength in facing and losing our worries. We may feel that they are temporary, and in time they will pass.

The process of surrender is powerful as it can free us from our worries and our anxieties. It can lighten our load. By surrendering, we have faith that we do not stand alone. By surrendering, we believe that there is something else that can help us to survive our heavy moments. We believe that there is something else to share our load.

The process of surrender allows us to release what we are holding so that our vital life energy can flow again. Our life energy can become stagnant and blocked by the worries and fears that we hold. When it becomes blocked, we struggle to live life as we are meant to, to live life in the now, and to feel supported in the now.

We have nothing to lose and everything to gain in surrendering and losing our worries. Our worries are a state of mind, created by something that has happened in the past that has caused us to fear our very own future. When we surrender our worries, we surrender our fear.

We can surrender knowing that much in life is out of our hands. We can surrender knowing that the fear we hold only serves to block us. We can surrender knowing that we are held in love and will return to love when we end our journey. We can surrender in love.

WEALTH: MONEY CAN BUY US GREED

There will be some in life that no matter what money or success they have, they will always be looking for more. They will always be looking for the next thing to have or to own. They will miss out on having because they are caught up in wanting.

Those who seem to have everything on the outside, may have little on the inside, yet those who have lost everything on the outside, may have gained everything on the inside. Sometimes, it is only by losing everything in life, that we can start to appreciate the simple life. We can start to take in the sun on our backs, the fresh air from the sea, the colour of autumn and the light from the moon and sun.

It is only by going through life without those moments that we can go back and really enjoy them, with new appreciation for their existence. It is only in the face of losing it all that we are born again, we can live again, and we can have new eyes for the world around us regardless of our financial status.

Those who are motivated in greed are not any happier than those who have less. In fact, those with less may be happier than those who have achieved financial success. The more that we have, the more we can complain as we look for and expect perfection.

Those, who want more may be looking to fill a void inside. A void inside can never be filled by something material on the outside. A void can never be bought. It can only be filled from the inside, for which material possessions play no part.

Money plays its part for avoiding financial stress. It can create temporary outer happiness, but it will never create lasting inner happiness. It can create superficial happiness, but we may find that the more we want, the more we compare ourselves to others. The more we compare, the more we judge and separate ourselves from each other and from the collective.

There are those who use their money and power for a higher good. There are those who have realised that by sharing their wealth, they grow their wealth, and, in the process, they empower others. They understand the reason for their money, is for it to be shared and not to be held. For it to be expressed outwards, not inwards. They understand that true wealth is found in helping and empowering others.

It is a common perception that money alone can give us true wealth, however it is only how we use it that can. When we start to share our wealth, it can bring us together, instead of tearing us apart. It is only in helping others that we receive the true happiness that comes with having money. It is only in sharing our wealth, that we will know the true power of our wealth, and the power in the collective acts towards each other.

HAPPINESS: FORGIVING THE PAST

We all make mistakes, and we all have past regrets. We all could have, should have and would have done things differently. We all have some level of darkness in our past, some darker than others. Sometimes instead of facing it, it is better to lock it away and continue to ignore it.

It is easier to ignore our feelings of regret and guilt from our past. It is easier to ignore the resentment and anger we hold towards others. Our past can come with the very feelings that hold us back from finding happiness in our lives. By ignoring it, we are held back from creating a brighter future.

It can be hard for us to open the door to the past and to let the memories come flooding out. It is difficult for us to process them, sit with them, welcome them, and forgive them. It is difficult for us to face the pain when we can keep it locked away for another day.

No matter how far we run or how far we travel, our past has an ironic way of showing up in our current life circumstances. Our past has a way of coming back to haunt us. It can keep re-appearing in different forms or scenarios, until we acknowledge it and are brave enough to face it, accept it and forgive it.

Our past is full of the mistakes we made, and others made. Our past will include suffering because of these mistakes but it comes a time when they need our forgiveness. In forgiveness we rise above our past, make peace with it and in doing so make peace with each other. In forgiveness, we find the true meaning of love and the true meaning of acceptance.

In facing our past, we face ourselves. We face the good, the bad, the hurt, the pain, the tears, and the heart ache. When we are ready to face it, we should never face it alone. We should seek the support of others. We should ask others for their love and their understanding in facing and forgiving our past.

We can face our past by breaking it up into pieces. We can face it little by little, step by step and if it becomes too much, we can face it another day. We can acknowledge our courage and strength in opening the door, if only to look. We should always take as much time as we need in forgiving what has gone before us.

In forgiving our past, we can begin the process of acceptance and understanding for our mistakes and those of others. We can begin the process of letting go. In accepting the past for what it was and forgiving others, we can move into the present. By moving into the present, we can find happiness. We can find happiness today when we make peace with our past. We can find happiness today in forgiveness.

LOVE: OUR FINAL DESTINATION

Like driving our cars, we all take a similar journey in life. We all share the same road towards a final destination. We all take an individual journey with a unique purpose. We all take the journey at our own pace. Some of us will wait and let others by, some cut across others and some will go along at a steady pace. Regardless of our pace, we all are all going towards a final destination. The only difference that stands between us is that some of us will arrive at our destination before others.

In life, the only thing we can know for sure is that when we reach our final destination, we can take nothing with us. We can only leave our legacy behind. We leave our legacy behind for our children, our grandchildren, our nieces, our nephews or for a wider audience. We leave a legacy behind that they can be proud of. We leave a legacy behind that they can grow and continue in love for us.

When we reach our final destination, we will realise that it is only the people we loved and loved us that will matter. We will realise that it is the memories that we have created together and the love that we have shared that will comfort and hold us in our final days. Everything else will fade into the background.

When we reach the end, we will realise that it will be our kindness and acts of generosity towards others for which we will be remembered. It will be for our love towards others that will matter the most. We will not be remembered for our financial status.

When we reach the end, we will realise that we could have left the world in a better place then how we found it. We will realise that we could have contributed to benefit future generations. We will reflect on the positive contribution we made towards others and our planet.

We should not wait until the end to realise all that could have been done today. We should not arrive at our final destination in regret. We can act today. We can give today. We can love today. We can act in love today. We can give back to a world that has given us so much. We can give back to our planet that needs it so much.

We can choose today how we would like to be remembered. We can choose to be remembered for what we gave and not for what we took. We can be remembered for our acts of generosity or acts of greed. We can be remembered for a positive and lasting legacy.

Our true legacy will be in the love and the memories that we leave behind. Our life is our chance to be remembered by others in love. It is our chance to leave a legacy to grow in love. It is our chance to love, to forgive and to live as we are meant to, together as one, together in love.

CHAPTER 12

A FINAL NOTE
ON HEALTH

I was nineteen when I was diagnosed with arthritis. It came on suddenly one morning and I could not get out of bed. It was a scary and lonely moment, losing my mobility like that. After the diagnosis, I started a course of steroids. The pain relief was short lived, and I soon started to suffer the side effects of taking medication. My mood and sleep were chaotic, and I had to give up my college and social life.

My twin sister who had also been diagnosed with the condition, decided to find an alternative solution for healing. I was equally as desperate to give anything but medication a go. I had no strong belief that energy healing could work but I was open to it and I was open to the possibilities of it.

The lady who performed this energy healing, gave my sister and I our lives back. It was not long after this healing, I had my social life back and I was free again. Free from pain, free to dance and free to live life again.

I was diagnosed with ulcerative colitis at the age of thirty. The diagnosis came shortly after I moved to Australia and at a time when I was looking to start a new life. It was also a time of massive stress and change in my life and although I had left Ireland behind, I took my emotional baggage with me.

After this diagnosis, I had no other option but to try medication again. I experienced many more side effects and I had long and lonely stays in the hospital. When I had a flare, it would knock me for months on end and I would lose myself physically and emotionally in the disease. I would lose my career because of it and in 2018, I had no other option but to return home.

My return home did not bring the healing that I had hoped for and I ended up in hospital again, on even stronger medication. I reached my lowest and loneliest point during these times. I was mentally and physically exhausted and I had nothing left within me to fight.

After reaching my lowest point, I had no more energy left to hold all the negativity I was holding inside. I started to make peace with what had been and my past. I started to forgive the disease. I decided to forgive all those who had hurt me, and I decided to surrender to something else. I decided to believe in something else and I decided to believe in me.

After a long internal healing process, I slowly started to turn a corner and I started to heal both physically and mentally. I started to look like me again. There was no one thing that happened, and there was no magic pill or cure. All I know for sure is that I changed my mind, and I changed my beliefs. I stated to take responsibility. I forgave, I loved, and I started to heal. I started to live again. My journey started to make sense to me and in a way my journey had just begun.

A FINAL NOTE
ON WEALTH

I became an engineer to make money and to be successful. My definition of success was to make my parents proud and to earn money. Engineers seemed to make good money and I was good at maths so at a career guidance session in school, I decided I would be an engineer.

I started off my career as a "success". I was earning good money and my parents were proud. I was taking on big challenges and succeeding. I was traveling the world with my work and I was respected. I could afford nice things, live in a nice apartment, and had a decent social life. On paper, I was wealthy but inside I was empty. I was lonely and I was sad.

I thought the answer to feeling lonely and sad was to relocate to Sydney. A new city and a new life could make me happy again and I could leave my unhappiness behind me. I could continue to earn good money and I would have plenty of places to spend it.

Initially this was true, and I had a great new life in Sydney. I made the best of friends and we had many a good night out. My loneliness was gone, and the change of scenery was doing me the world of good. I was finally enjoying life, that was until my health got in the way. That was until I realised, I had no wealth without it, and I had no life without it.

On the days I was confined to bed and struggled to eat, I would have given anything to have my appetite again. On the nights I did not sleep, I would have given anything to have my sleep again. On the days when I was lonely in bed, I would have given anything to see my friends again. It was all gone and in losing it I started to realise the true meaning of wealth and it had nothing to do with money.

I realised that I needed money to pay the bills and I needed it to survive but I did not need it to feel wealthy. My health was my wealth, my friends were my wealth, and my food was my wealth. Everything I had taken for granted before was my wealth. I already had it, but I did not know I was wealthy. It took the disease to remind me to be grateful for it when it did return.

I live my life today with little financially, but I have everything else in abundance. I have a peaceful home and I am surrounded by nature. I am surrounded by unconditional love given to me by my dogs and my partner. I feel and experience true love every day and I feel wealthier inside than I ever did before.

I am wealthy because I have been given a second chance at life and a second chance at love and I am willing to take it. I am willing to live my life to the full and I am willing to love to the full. I am willing to share my wealth with others, and that is my life journey so far, my life lessons so far, and my belief that no matter how dark our days are, that brighter ones lie ahead.

A FINAL NOTE ON HAPPINESS

I did not find out what true happiness meant until I could forgive and accept my past. Until I could forgive my past, I was holding anger inside. Until I could accept my past, I was holding resentment inside.

Forgiveness and acceptance cannot come over night. It takes work and it takes patience. It takes pain and tears to forgive those that have hurt us. It is by no means easy, to forgive those we have loved and who have not loved us back. It takes courage to open up the door and heal our past.

I was stuck in past resentment which was preventing me from living my life in the present moment. I was blocking my life energy and holding on to memories that no longer served me. It was done and in the past, but I was holding it as if it was protecting me from getting hurt again.

When I reached my lowest point, it did not seem to matter anymore what anyone else had said or done. It did not seem to make sense to hold on to it anymore and it felt right to start to forgive and let go. I realised I had to stop waiting for those around me to love me or to save me. I had no choice but to start loving myself.

As I started to forgive and let go, the part of me that used to be happy, started to come back and show her light again to me. She wanted to come out and play and I let her. She wanted to laugh and I let her. I slowly started not to take life so seriously and not take myself so seriously.

Living on the lighter side of life suited me. It was easier to live that way than hold on to worry and stress. I started to laugh at myself and my situation and it became easier to deal with. It helped me to turn the situation around. I was done crying and decided it was time to laugh instead. In laughter, I lightened my load.

As I stated to forgive and accept my past, I started to love again. I had thought I had loved before, and I had spoken of love but I had never truly felt it. When I did feel it, it came fast, and it came strong. I now make time to love myself and make my decisions for me and not to keep other people happy.

By loving myself, I can love others and I can help others. By forgiving and accepting my past, I can move on with my life. I can leave it behind for what it was and not what I wanted it to be. I do not need to feel fear of the past and I can embrace my future.

Finding our inner happiness is a lifelong journey. There is no single moment that we reach when it is all there. It comes and goes, in waves, like the ocean, some days stronger than others, some days it recedes, and some days it is still. Each state is temporary, our lives are temporary but with love and forgiveness we can make a lasting impact. We can be happy and make others happy in the process.

A FINAL NOTE ON LOVE

I found out what love was at my lowest point in life and it took pain to know what real love was. To see it in its entirety I had to go through the pain, and I had to suffer. I had not seen it like that before. The love before was superficial on the surface. The love before was conditional. The love at my lowest shone brightly, it was deeper, and it had more meaning. Someone was showing me that they loved me at my weakest, their actions were speaking for themselves and I felt it strongly.

When you rushed to be by my side when I got the bad news, when you tucked me up in bed, when you put my socks on, when you cooked for hours on end, when you changed my bed sheets, when you held my hand and sat with me until I could sleep, you showed me what true love was. You showed me that our love in the good times was easy but our love in the hard times was real.

You could see past the physical and you could still see me. You saw the beauty in me when I could not. You supported my decisions and understood my pain. You loved me at my lowest and you believed in me at my weakest. You never stopped loving me even when I stopped loving myself. You never gave up on our love or our future. You held it safe, and you protected it.

If it had not been for the illness, I would not have known love fully and I would not have known you. It showed me your strength, your character, your patience, and the true meaning of in sickness and in health. You were living our vows even though we had yet to take them. You were standing up to the responsibility of me, and of us. You were putting your life on hold for me, and you were willing to wait. You were willing to still love when everything else faded away.

If it were not for those times, I would not have appreciated the present and our future ahead of us. I treasure every day now because of it. I stop, I look, I enjoy, I take it all in. When I spend time with you and our dogs, it melts my heart like no other. When we walk together in nature, I take it all in. I take it all in and I am grateful. I am grateful of the beauty that surrounds me. I am grateful to hold your hand. I am grateful to walk. I am grateful to love and be loved.

The illness was my wake-up call. A call to see life again through new eyes and to live life again from the heart. A call to feel love again and to treasure each moment I have with those that I love. A call to know love again through forgiveness and acceptance of what was and what is.

To love and feel love is a gift, and we can all give love for as long as we have left. For in the end, it will be only love that will last. It is only love that survives all else and it is only love that will matter. When all is said and done, it is only our love that we will remember, love for each other, love for ourselves, and love for our life.

A FINAL NOTE FOR YOU

The same creator created us all in love and the same creator holds us all in love. When we look at the ocean, the trees, the sky, and the birds, we can see the beauty within each. The same beauty is within you and we have all been created in the same beauty.

Never give up on yourself and never stop looking again for the beauty inside you for it is there, waiting to shine brightly again. It is there waiting to know you again. It is there waiting to show you love again.

You are worth health, wealth, happiness, and love. You are worth all that life has to offer and you are worth your dreams and your desires. When the days seem dark and life gets heavy, take a break, to rest and to slow down. Take a break to breathe again.

With each new day, comes a new beginning and comes a new hope. With each new day, comes a new light, that we can start again, we can forgive, and we can love again. Each new day is a day to live our lives as we were meant to, as a beautiful soul, grounded in love, supported in love, and eternally held in love, until we return again.

WE ARE ONE

We are one
We are connected
Connected by our light

We are one
We are a collective
A collective by our light

We are one
We are love
Love by our light

We are one, Just one
One Journey, One light
One love,
One home

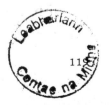

117

ACKNOWLEDGEMENTS

My own journey has been supported by many people and it continues with many more. I would like to thank each of you for being with me either past or present, and to the many more adventures that lie ahead.

For my parents, my sisters, and my nephew

For my uncles, aunties and cousins

For my second parents

For my grandparents

For the beautiful souls that have passed

For my friends

For my teachers

For my healers

For the doctors and nurses

For the strangers that showed me kindness

For Jack, Cora and for my Love, Des

Printed in Great Britain
by Amazon